I0693902

SAY NO

TO

CANCER

DEDICATED

TO ALL

LIVING SOUL

ACKNOWLEGEMENT

All praise and adoration is due to nobody except

almighty God the lord of mankind. I praise him and

glorified him for is protections and blessings over

me so far. And also for giving me opportunities to

create this small work, for the benefit of my

readers. I am also indebted to my late father for his

tremendous efforts to make my education

successful. May his gentle soul continue to rest in

perfect peace till eternity (amen). And also to my

great mother for her intensive supports on very

steps I take. May she live long to eat the fruit of her

labor. This work would not have seen the light of

the day if not for the prayers, patronage and

encouragement of my readers. I thank you all, may

almighty God in his infinity mercy continue and

protect every one of us (amen).

CONTENTS

<u>**_Section 1_**</u>**_: Figuring out Malignant growth_**

Malignant growth is an illness portrayed by the uncontrolled development and spread of strange cells in the body. There are various sorts of disease, each with its own arrangement of side effects, risk elements, and treatment choices.

Sound cells in the body develop and isolate in a methodical way to supplant old or harmed cells. Be that as it may, when cells become unusual and start to develop and isolate wildly, they can shape a mass of tissue called a growth. Not all growths are dangerous; growths that are not carcinogenic are called harmless cancers, while destructive cancers are called threatening cancers.

Disease can foster in any piece of the body and can spread to different pieces of the body through the circulation system or lymphatic framework. The spread of disease from its unique site to different pieces of the body is called metastasis.

The specific reasons for malignant growth are not completely perceived, however research has recognized a few gamble factors that can improve an individual's probability of fostering the illness. These gamble factors include:

Hereditary transformations: Certain changes in qualities can build the gamble of creating disease.
Age: Malignant growth is more normal in more seasoned grown-ups.
Ecological elements: Openness to specific natural variables, for example, tobacco smoke, radiation, and certain synthetic substances, can expand the gamble of creating malignant growth.
Way of life factors: Certain way of life factors, like a less than stellar eating routine, absence of active work, and exorbitant liquor utilization, can build the gamble of creating disease.

Early discovery and therapy are critical in the administration of malignant growth. Therapy choices for malignant growth incorporate a medical procedure, radiation treatment, chemotherapy, and designated treatment. The decision of therapy relies upon the kind and phase of disease, as well as the singular's general wellbeing and inclinations.

In the following section, we will examine systems for disease avoidance and early discovery.

Section 2: Avoidance Systems

While there is no surefire method for forestalling malignant growth, there are a few techniques that can lessen the gamble of fostering the sickness. These techniques include:

Sound way of life decisions: Taking on a solid way of life can fundamentally diminish the gamble of creating disease. This incorporates keeping a solid weight, eating a sound eating routine, participating in standard active work, staying away from tobacco items, and restricting liquor utilization.

Sun wellbeing: Openness to bright (UV) radiation from the sun and tanning beds can expand the gamble of skin malignant growth. Safeguarding the skin from UV radiation by wearing defensive apparel, looking for shade, and utilizing sunscreen can diminish the gamble of skin disease.

Inoculations: Immunizations can safeguard against specific sorts of disease causing infections, for example, the human papillomavirus (HPV) and hepatitis B infection (HBV).

Screening and early discovery: Screening tests can distinguish disease at a beginning phase, when it is more treatable. Suggested screening tests shift contingent upon the sort of malignant growth and a singular's age and chance elements.

Natural mindfulness: Monitoring ecological variables that can build the gamble of disease, like openness to specific synthetics, can assist people with doing whatever it may take to decrease their openness.

Hereditary testing and advising: A few people might be at expanded chance of creating disease because of acquired hereditary transformations. Hereditary testing and advising can assist people with understanding their gamble and come to informed conclusions about counteraction and screening.

It is critical to take note of that while these procedures can lessen the gamble of creating malignant growth, they don't ensure avoidance. It is likewise essential to keep looking for proper clinical consideration and screenings, regardless of whether you are following these counteraction systems.

In the following section, we will examine the significance of early discovery and the different screening tests accessible for various sorts of disease.

<u>**Section 3**</u>: **Early Discovery and Screening**

Early location of malignant growth is critical for effective treatment and further developed results. Screening tests are utilized to distinguish malignant growth before side effects create, taking into account prior finding and treatment.

There are a few different screening tests accessible for various kinds of malignant growth. The suggested screening tests fluctuate contingent upon an individual's age, sex, and hazard factors for explicit sorts of disease.

Here are the absolute most normal screening tests:

<u>**Mammography**</u>: A mammogram is a X-beam of the bosom tissue used to distinguish bosom disease. The American Disease Society suggests that ladies at normal gamble of bosom malignant growth have a mammogram at

regular intervals between the ages of 50 and 74.

Pap smear: A Pap smear is a test that inspects cells from the cervix for irregularities that might demonstrate cervical malignant growth. The American Disease Society suggests that ladies start having Pap spreads at age 21 and proceed with at regular intervals until age 29. After age 30, ladies ought to have a Pap smear and human papillomavirus (HPV) test at regular intervals or a Pap smear alone like clockwork.

Colonoscopy: A colonoscopy is a test that looks at the colon for polyps or indications of colorectal malignant growth. The American Disease Society suggests that people at normal gamble of colorectal malignant growth start screening at age 45 with either a colonoscopy like clockwork, a waste immunochemical test (FIT) consistently, or a stool DNA test at regular intervals.

Prostate-explicit antigen (public service announcement) test: A public service announcement test is a blood test used to recognize prostate disease in men. The American Malignant growth Society suggests that men talk about the expected advantages and dangers of public service announcement testing with their primary care physician beginning at age 50, or prior for those at higher gamble.

Skin assessment: A skin assessment is utilized to recognize skin malignant growth. The American Disease Society suggests that people perform month to month self-assessments of their skin and look for proficient assessments for any dubious moles or sores.

It is vital to converse with a specialist about individual gamble factors and suggested screening tests. Early recognition and incite therapy can essentially expand the possibilities of effective disease treatment and recuperation.

In the following section, we will examine the different therapy choices accessible for malignant growth.

<u>Section 4</u>: Option and Reciprocal Treatments

While customary therapies like a medical procedure, chemotherapy, and radiation treatment are the standard techniques for treating malignant growth, many individuals likewise go to option and correlative treatments for extra help during their disease process. Elective treatments are utilized rather than regular medicines, while reciprocal treatments are utilized notwithstanding ordinary medicines.

Here are a few other option and correlative treatments ordinarily utilized for disease:

<u>**Needle therapy**</u>: Needle therapy includes the addition of fine needles into explicit focuses on the body to animate mending and ease torment. A few examinations propose that needle therapy might assist with mitigating the symptoms of chemotherapy and radiation treatment.

Home grown medication: Natural cures are regular items produced using plants, and certain individuals use them to help their insusceptible framework during disease treatment. Notwithstanding, it is critical to take note of that home grown cures can cooperate with chemotherapy drugs and different prescriptions, so it is fundamental for converse with a specialist prior to utilizing them.

Contemplation and unwinding strategies: Reflection, yoga, and other unwinding procedures can assist with decreasing pressure, uneasiness, and gloom, and work on by and large prosperity during malignant growth treatment.

Dietary enhancements: Certain individuals take dietary enhancements like nutrients, minerals, and other regular items to help their safe framework and diminish the gamble of disease. Notwithstanding, it is critical to converse with a specialist prior to accepting any enhancements as they might connect with chemotherapy drugs and different meds.

Rub treatment: Back rub treatment can assist with decreasing nervousness and stress, alleviate torment and weariness, and work on generally prosperity during disease treatment.

It is critical to take note of that other option and integral treatments are not a substitute for customary malignant growth treatment. It is fundamental to examine any other option or correlative treatments with a specialist to guarantee they are protected and don't disrupt customary treatment.

In the following section, we will examine the different traditional therapy choices accessible for malignant growth.

<u>*Section 5: Adapting to Malignant growth*</u>

A disease determination can be overpowering and sincerely testing. Adapting to malignant growth includes figuring out how to deal with the physical, close to home, and mental impacts of the sickness.

Here are a few ways to adapt to disease:

<u>Look for help</u>: Converse with loved ones about your analysis and treatment plan. Joining a malignant growth support gathering or looking for proficient directing can likewise offer important help.

<u>Remain informed</u>: Advance however much you can about your disease analysis and treatment choices. This can assist you with feeling more in charge and better ready to come to informed conclusions about your consideration.

<u>Practice taking care of oneself</u>: Deal with your physical and profound prosperity by eating a solid eating routine, getting sufficient rest, and participating in ordinary active work. Practice unwinding strategies, for example, contemplation or yoga to diminish pressure.

Speak with your medical services group: Remain nearby with your primary care physicians and attendants about your side effects, aftereffects, and concerns. They can give direction and backing as you explore your treatment.

Keep an uplifting perspective: An inspirational perspective and disposition can assist you with adapting to the difficulties of malignant growth treatment. Remain confident and center around the things that give you pleasure and satisfaction.

Acknowledge help: Don't hesitate for even a moment to request help or acknowledge help from others. Companions, family, and local area assets can offer viable help like transportation or feast conveyance.

Adapting to malignant growth can be a long and troublesome excursion, yet with the right help and assets, dealing with the physical and close to home impacts of the disease is conceivable. Make sure to take it each day in turn and to connect for help when required.

In the last section, we will examine the significance of disease research and the most recent headways in malignant growth treatment.

<u>*Section* 6</u>*: Facing everyday life After Disease*

Subsequent to finishing disease treatment, many individuals experience a scope of feelings, from help and appreciation to uneasiness and vulnerability about what's on the horizon. Facing everyday life after disease includes changing in accordance with another typical and tracking down lifestyle choices a solid and satisfying life.

Here are a few hints for life after malignant growth:

<u>**Circle back to your medical services group**</u>: It is essential to proceed with normal subsequent meetings with your PCPs to screen your wellbeing and distinguish any expected repeat or secondary effects from therapy.

<u>**Settle on solid way of life decisions**</u>: A sound way of life can assist with lessening the gamble of malignant growth repeat and work on in general prosperity. This incorporates keeping a

solid eating regimen, taking part in normal actual work, and keeping away from tobacco and exorbitant liquor utilization.

Track down help: Joining a disease survivorship gathering or looking for proficient guiding can offer significant help as you explore life after malignant growth. Conversing with different survivors can likewise assist you with feeling less alone and give important bits of knowledge into survival techniques.

Center around taking care of oneself: Set aside a few minutes for taking care of oneself exercises that give you pleasure and assist with decreasing pressure, like reflection, yoga, or investing energy in nature.

Put forth reasonable objectives: Defining reachable objectives can assist you with recapturing a feeling of control and reason after malignant growth treatment. Begin with little objectives and move gradually up to greater ones as you recover strength and certainty.

Embrace appreciation: Rehearsing appreciation can assist with moving your concentration from the provokes of malignant growth treatment to the positive parts of life. Take time every day to ponder the things you are thankful for and to offer your thanks to other people.

Facing everyday life after disease can be a difficult and remunerating venture. With the right help, assets, and an inspirational perspective, carrying on with a satisfying and solid life after cancer is conceivable.

<u>**Section 7: Support and Mindfulness**</u>

Backing and mindfulness are basic parts in the battle against disease. By supporting for better disease counteraction, therapy, and examination, and bringing issues to light about the significance of malignant growth anticipation and early recognition, we can diminish the effect of disease on people and networks.

Here are far to engage in disease support and mindfulness:

<u>**Take part in disease related occasions**</u>: Numerous associations have occasions like strolls, runs, and pledge drives to bring issues to light and assets for malignant growth examination and patient help. Partaking in these occasions can assist with bringing issues to light and support for the purpose.

<u>**Engage in backing endeavors**</u>: Promotion endeavors include upholding for strategies and regulation that help disease anticipation, treatment, and examination. Joining a

promotion bunch or reaching your chosen authorities can assist with having an effect in the battle against malignant growth.

Teach others: Sharing data about malignant growth avoidance and early location with family, companions, and your local area can assist with bringing issues to light and urge others to find proactive ways to diminish their disease risk.

Support disease research: Giving to malignant growth research associations or partaking in clinical preliminaries can assist with supporting the improvement of new disease medicines and treatments.

Volunteer: Chipping in at malignant growth support associations or medical clinics can offer important help to disease patients and their families and assist with bringing issues to light about the effect of disease.

By engaging in malignant growth support and mindfulness endeavors, we can all have an effect in the battle against disease. Together, we can attempt to lessen the weight of malignant growth and further develop results for those impacted by this infection.

All in all, malignant growth is a mind boggling illness that influences a great many individuals around the world. While progress has been made in disease counteraction, treatment, and examination, there is still a lot of work to be finished. By becoming backers for change and bringing issues to light about the significance of disease anticipation and early identification, we can cooperate to decrease the effect of malignant growth on people and networks.

www.ingramcontent.com/pod-product-compliance
Lightning Source LLC
Chambersburg PA
CBHW081545250726
48659CB00009B/3086